# The Low Carb Diet Guide

Including a Weight Loss Diet Guide and 25
Delicious Recipes

## Disclaimer and Terms of Use:

Effort has been made to ensure that the information in this book is accurate and complete, however, the author and the publisher do not warrant the accuracy of the information, text and graphics contained within the book due to the rapidly changing nature of science, research, known and unknown facts and internet. The Author and the publisher do not hold any responsibility for errors, omissions or contrary interpretation of the subject matter herein. This book is presented solely for motivational and informational purposes only.

# Table of Contents

# Introduction

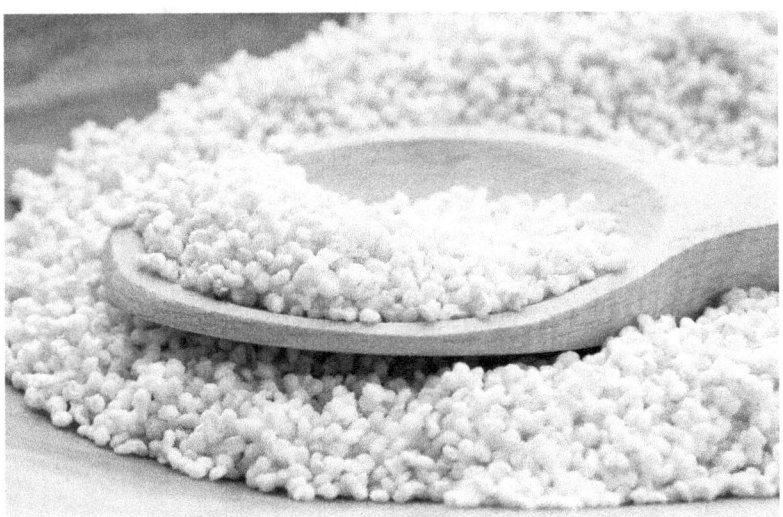

One of the most popular modern diets is the Low Carb Diet. This diet is exactly what it sounds like – a diet that is low in carbohydrates, particularly processed grains and starchy vegetables. This type of diet doesn't just limit your intake of carbs, it also places an emphasis on foods that are high in both protein and fat. Sometimes the Low Carb Diet is called the Low Carb High Fat Diet (LCHF). The most common use for the Low Carb Diet is for weight loss – decreasing your carb intake while increase your protein intake can help you to burn more calories and lose weight. If you are thinking about giving the Low Carb Diet a try, this book is the perfect place to start. Here you will find an introduction to the diet, a list of foods to eat and avoid, and a collection of 25 delicious low-carb recipes.

# About the Low Carb Diet for Weight Loss

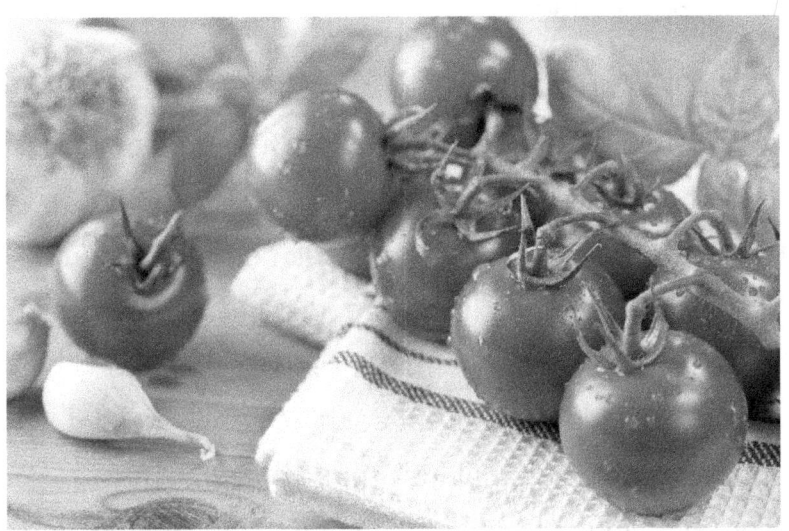

The Low-Carb Diet is a diet that limits your intake of carbohydrates, particularly high-glycemic carbohydrates, in order to help you lose weight. This diet doesn't just help you lose weight, however – it can also help you to improve your overall health and eating habits which, in turn, might help you experience relief from the symptoms of chronic diseases. To follow the Low Carb Diet you should limit your intake of high-carbohydrate foods like grains, fruits, legumes, and dairy products. Certain nuts, seeds, and vegetables also contain carbohydrates. This diet requires you to reduce your intake of carbohdyrates while focusing instead on protein-right and high-fat foods.

The recommendations for the Low Carb Diet advocate for a daily limit of 60 to 130 grams of carbohydrate – this equates to about 240 to 520 calories. The rest of your daily calories should come from protein and fat. If you are trying to lose weight on the Low Carb Diet you should keep track of the number of calories you eat each day, making sure that you burn more calories than you consume. Focusing your diet on lean proteins, healthy fats, and low-carb vegetables will help you to meet your weight loss goals. To help you get started on the Low Carb Diet, consult the food lists below:

## Foods to Avoid on the Diet

- Wheat
- Barley
- Rye
- Triticale
- Spelt
- Bread
- Pasta
- Baked goods
- Fruit juice
- Soft drinks
- Agave
- Ice cream
- Candy

- Soybean oil
- Sunflower oil
- Corn oil
- Canola oil
- Grape seed oil
- Artificial sweetener
- Diet products
- Low-fat foods
- Processed foods

## Foods to Eat on the Diet

- Beef
- Pork
- Chicken
- Turkey
- Lamb
- Fresh fish
- Shellfish
- Eggs
- Fresh vegetables
- Apples
- Orange
- Pears
- Blueberries
- Strawberries
- Almonds
- Walnuts
- Brazil nuts
- Pine nuts
- Pecans
- Sunflower seeds
- Flaxseed
- Sesame seeds
- Chia seeds
- Cheese
- Butter
- Heavy cream

- Milk
- Yogurt
- Coconut oil
- Butter

- Lard
- Olive oil
- Avocado

- Almond flour
- Coconut flour

## Foods to Eat in Moderation

- Rice
- Oats
- Quinoa
- Amaranth

- Tapioca
- Lentils
- Dried beans
- Sweet potatoes

- Potatoes
- Dark chocolate
- Wine

Now that you understand the basics of the Low Carb Diet you are ready to get started! Consult the lists above to clean out and restock your pantry and then pick a recipe to try.

# Low Carb Diet Recipes

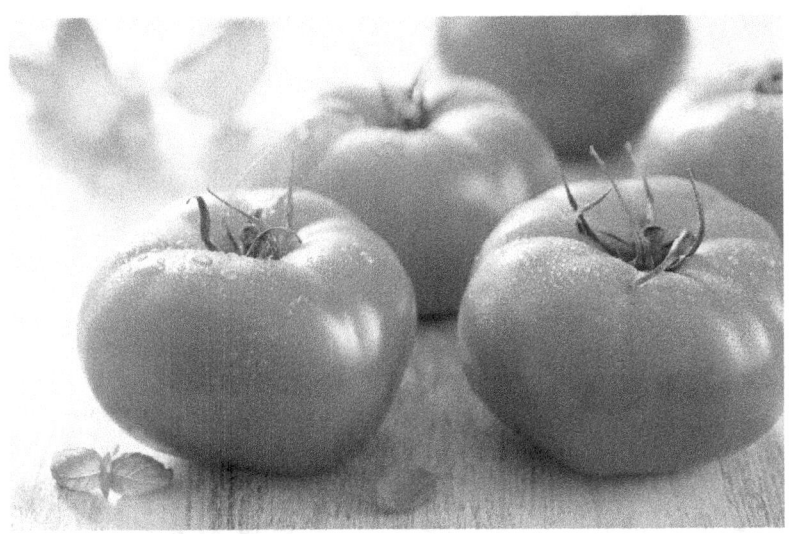

## <u>Recipes Included in this Book</u>:

Mushroom and Onion Omelet

Blueberry Yogurt Smoothie

Almond Flour Cinnamon Muffins

Broccoli Cheddar Egg Cups

Strawberry Almond Smoothie

Pumpkin Walnut Muffins

Mixed Vegetable Frittata

Avocado Lime Smoothie with Walnut

Carrot Ginger Soup

Red Cabbage Carrot Slaw

Tomato Basil Soup

Chopped Cobb Salad

Cream of Mushroom Soup

Spinach Bacon and Egg Salad

Pumpkin Cinnamon Soup

Grilled Salmon with Mango Sauce

Chicken Cordon-Bleu

Grilled Blue Cheese Burgers

Slow-Cooker Beef Bourguignon

Easy Homemade Meatloaf

Chocolate No-Bake Cookies

Strawberry Sorbet

Avocado Chocolate Pudding

Meringue Cookies

Cherry Granita

## *Mushroom and Onion Omelet*

**Servings**: 1

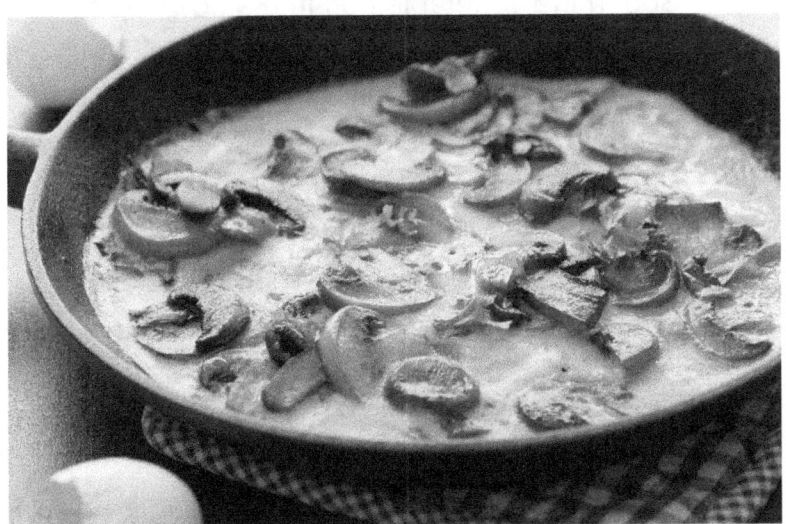

**Ingredients**:

2 teaspoons olive oil, divided

½ cup diced mushrooms

2 tablespoons diced yellow onion

1 clove garlic, minced

2 large eggs

1 tablespoon sliced green onion

Salt and pepper to taste

**Instructions**:

1. Heat 1 teaspoon of oil in a small skillet over medium heat.

2. Add the mushroom, onion, and garlic – cook for 3 to 4 minutes until tender.
3. Spoon the vegetables off into a bowl then reheat the skillet with the remaining oil.
4. Whisk together the egg, green onion, salt and pepper then pour into the skillet.
5. Cook for 2 minutes or until the egg is almost set.
6. Spoon the vegetables over half the omelet.
7. Fold the empty half of the omelet over the filling and cook for another minute or until the egg is set.

## *Blueberry Yogurt Smoothie*

**Servings**: 1 to 2

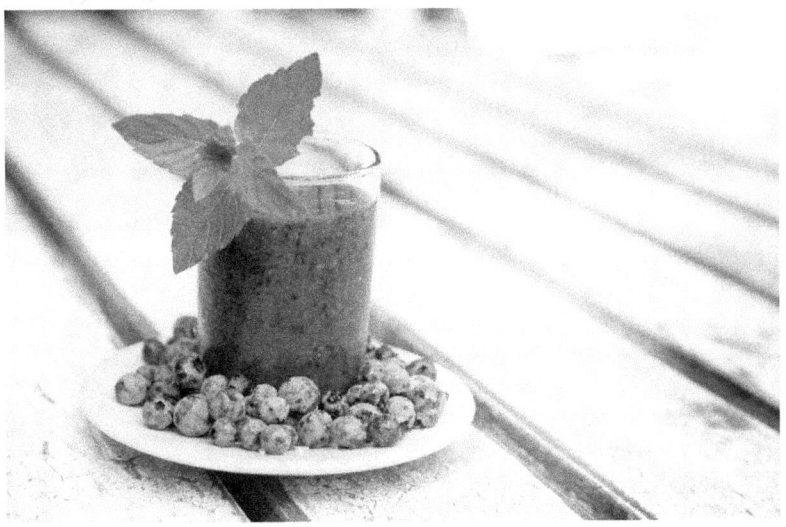

**Ingredients**:

2 cups frozen blueberries

1 small frozen banana, peeled and sliced

1 cup nonfat Greek yogurt

½ cup skim milk

2 tablespoons fresh mint

1 teaspoon honey

**Instructions**:

1. Combine the ingredients in a high-speed blender.

2.  Blend for 30 to 60 seconds until smooth and well combined.
3.  Divide the smoothie among two glasses and serve immediately.

## *Almond Flour Cinnamon Muffins*

**Servings**: 12

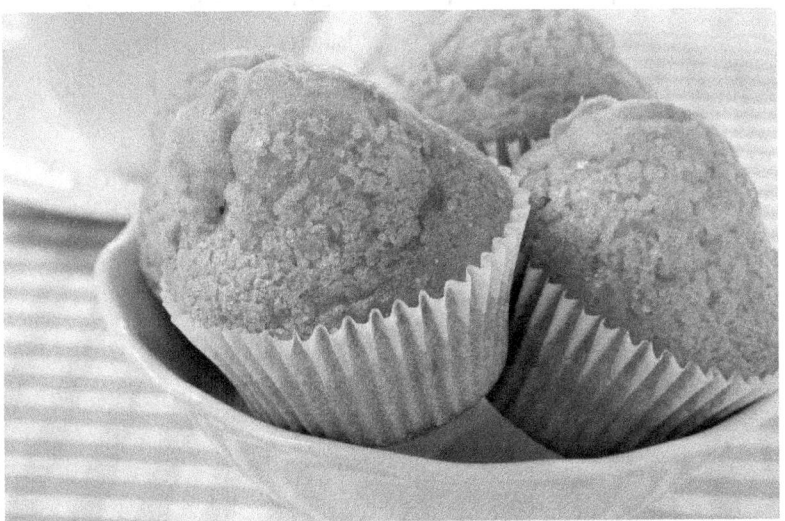

**Ingredients**:

2 cups blanched almond flour

1 teaspoon ground cinnamon

¾ teaspoon baking soda

¼ teaspoon salt

2 large eggs, whisked

1 cup unsweetened applesauce

1/3 cup raw honey

3 tablespoons melted coconut oil

**Instructions**:

1. Preheat the oven to 350°F (180°C) and line a muffin pan with paper liners.
2. Combine the dry ingredients in a mixing bowl.
3. In a separate bowl, whisk together the wet ingredients – stir the dry ingredients into the wet in small batches.
4. Spoon the batter into the muffin pan, filling the cups about 2/3 full.
5. Bake for 20 to 25 minutes until a knife inserted in the center comes out clean.
6. Cool the muffins for 5 minutes in the pan then turn out onto a wire rack to cool completely.

## *Broccoli Cheddar Egg Cups*

**Servings**: 12

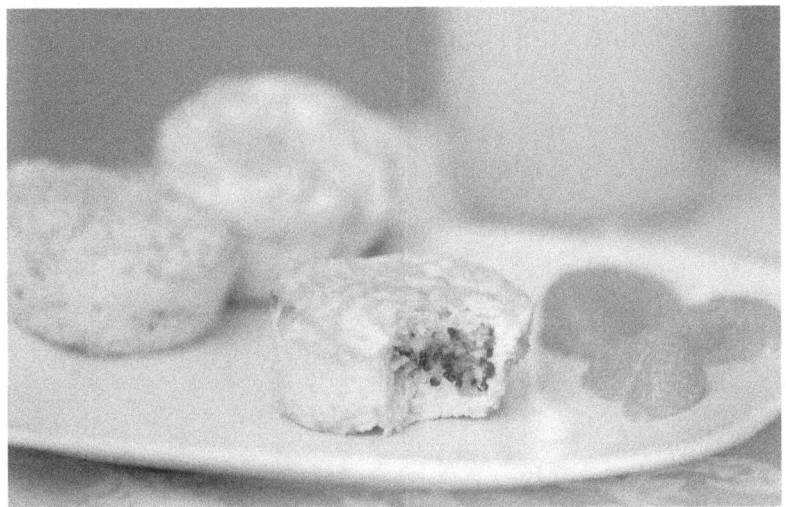

**Ingredients**:

12 large eggs

¼ cup skim milk

½ cup diced yellow onion

Salt and pepper to taste

1 ½ cups chopped broccoli

½ cup shredded cheddar

**Instructions**:

1. Preheat the oven to 350°F (180°C) and grease a muffin pan with cooking spray
2. Whisk together the eggs, milk, onion, salt and pepper.

3. Divide the broccoli among the cups and fill with the egg mixture.
4. Sprinkle with cheese and bake for 20 to 25 minutes until cooked through.

## Strawberry Almond Smoothie

**Servings**: 1 to 2

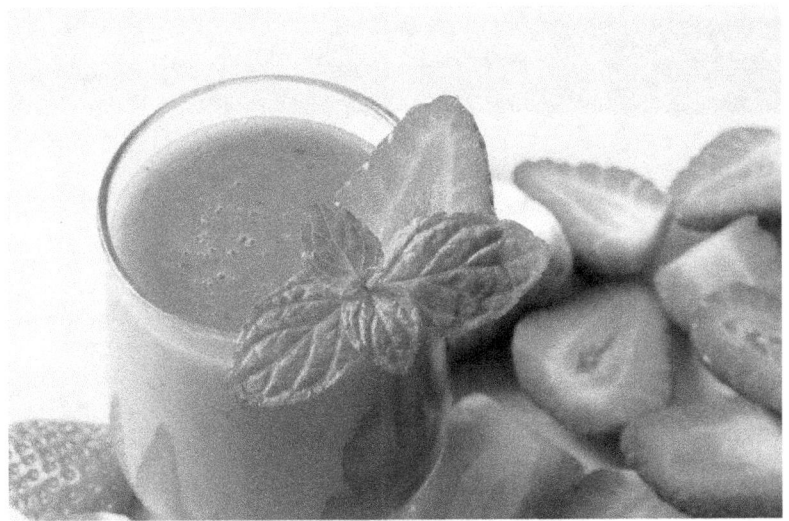

**Ingredients**:

1 ½ cups frozen strawberries

1 medium frozen banana, peeled and sliced

1 cup unsweetened almond milk

½ cup plain nonfat yogurt

2 tablespoons chopped almonds

**Instructions**:

1. Combine the ingredients in a high-speed blender.
2. Blend for 30 to 60 seconds until smooth and well combined.

3. Divide the smoothie among two glasses and serve immediately.

## *Pumpkin Walnut Muffins*

**Servings**: 12

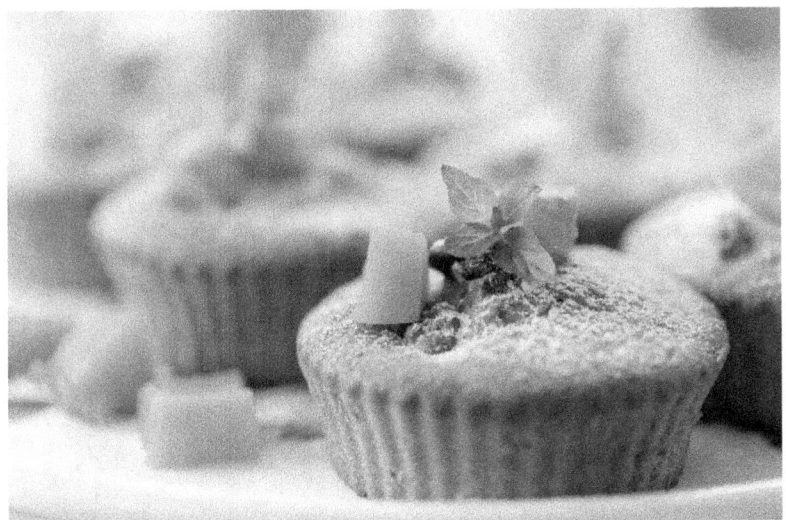

**Ingredients**:

2 cups blanched almond flour

1 teaspoon ground cinnamon

¾ teaspoon baking soda

½ teaspoon ground nutmeg

¼ teaspoon salt

2 large eggs, whisked

1 cup pumpkin puree

1/3 cup raw honey

3 tablespoons melted coconut oil

**Instructions**:

1. Preheat the oven to 350°F (180°C) and line a muffin pan with paper liners.
2. Combine the dry ingredients in a mixing bowl.
3. In a separate bowl, whisk together the wet ingredients – stir the dry ingredients into the wet in small batches.
4. Spoon the batter into the muffin pan, filling the cups about 2/3 full.
5. Bake for 20 to 25 minutes until a knife inserted in the center comes out clean.
6. Cool the muffins for 5 minutes in the pan then turn out onto a wire rack to cool completely.

## *Mixed Vegetable Frittata*

**Servings**: 6

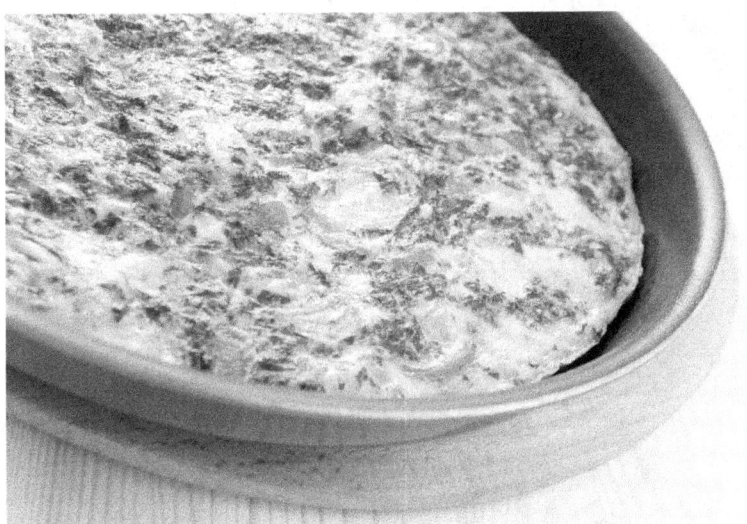

**Ingredients**:

1 tablespoon coconut oil

8 large eggs, beaten

1 small yellow onion, chopped

2 cups sliced mushrooms

1 small red pepper, cored and diced

½ cup skim milk

Salt and pepper to taste

1 ½ cups chopped spinach

**Instructions**:

1. Heat the oil in a large skillet over medium heat.
2. Add the onion, mushrooms and red pepper – cook for 4 to 6 minutes until tender.
3. Beat together the eggs, milk, salt and pepper then pour into the skillet.
4. Stir in the spinach then cook, covered, on low heat for 8 to 10 minutes until the eggs are almost set.
5. Turn off the heat then cover and let rest for 5 to 10 minutes until set.

## *Avocado Lime Smoothie with Walnut*

**Servings**: 1 to 2

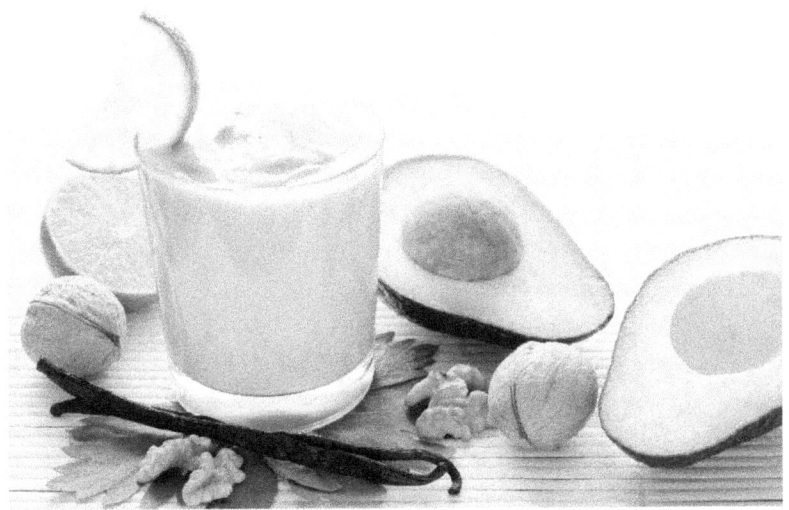

**Ingredients**:

1 large frozen banana, peeled and sliced

1 small ripe avocado, pitted and chopped

1 cup skim milk, cold

½ cup nonfat Greek yogurt

2 tablespoons chopped walnuts

1 teaspoon honey

**Instructions**:

1. Combine the ingredients in a high-speed blender.

2. Blend for 30 to 60 seconds until smooth and well combined.
3. Divide the smoothie among two glasses and serve immediately.

## *Carrot Ginger Soup*

**Servings**: 4 to 6

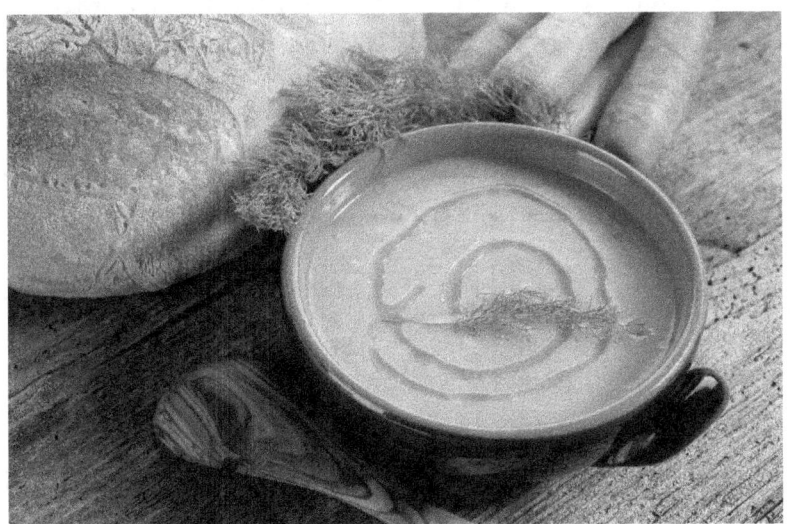

**Ingredients**:

1 tablespoon olive oil

1 ¼ lbs. chopped carrots

1 medium white onion, chopped

1 large Yukon gold potato, peeled and chopped

1 tablespoon fresh minced ginger

4 cups vegetable broth

2 teaspoons fresh lemon juice

Salt and pepper to taste

**Instructions**:

1. Heat the oil in a Dutch oven over medium-high heat.
2. Stir in the carrots, onion, potato and ginger – cook for 6 to 8 minutes until the onions are tender.
3. Add the remaining ingredients and stir well.
4. Bring to a boil then reduce heat and simmer for 25 minutes until the vegetables are tender.
5. Remove from heat and puree the soup using an immersion blender.
6. Season with salt and pepper to taste then serve hot.

## *Red Cabbage Carrot Slaw*

**Servings**: 8

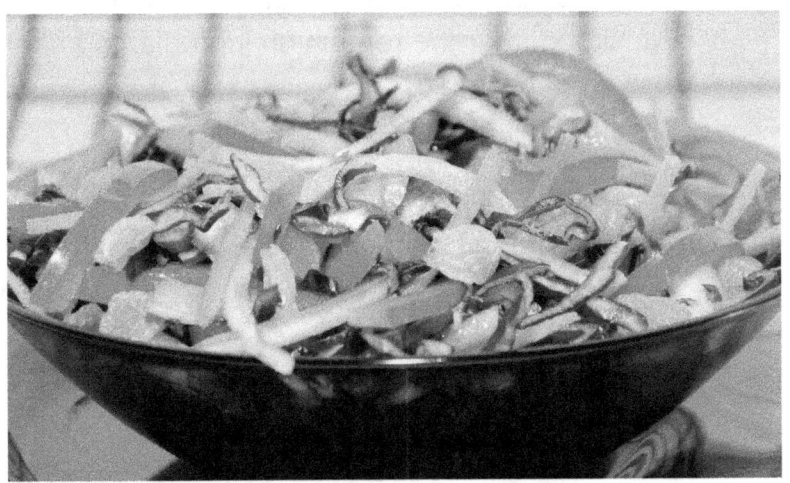

**Ingredients**:

5 cups sliced red cabbage

2 ½ cups grated or shredded carrot

1 small red onion, sliced thin

1 medium red pepper, cored and sliced thin

½ cup white wine vinegar

1 tablespoon honey

1 clove minced garlic

Pinch dried oregano

Salt and pepper to taste

**Instructions**:

1. Combine the cabbage, carrots, red onion and red pepper in a salad bowl.
2. Toss the vegetables until well combined.
3. Whisk together the remaining ingredients and toss with the salad.
4. Chill the salad until ready to serve.

## *Tomato Basil Soup*

**Servings**: 4 to 6

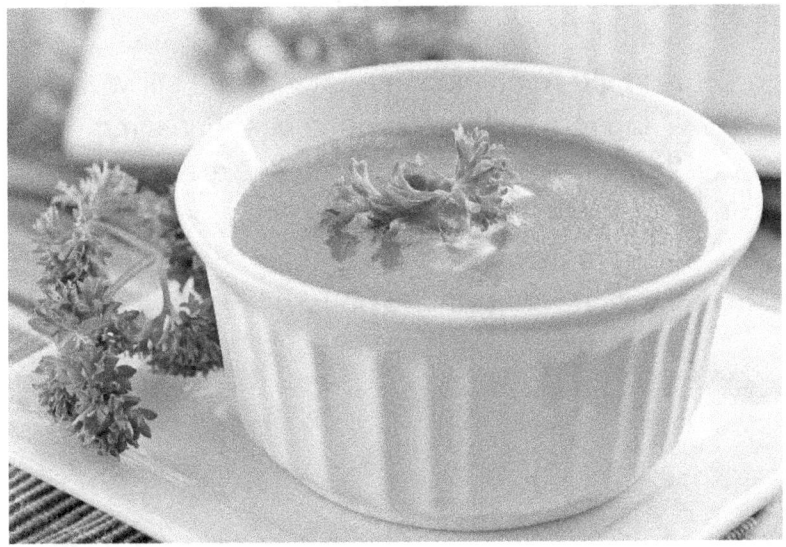

**Ingredients**:

1 tablespoon olive oil

1 tablespoon minced garlic

1 large yellow onion, chopped

3 (14.5 ounce) cans diced tomatoes

3 cups vegetable broth

1 cup fresh chopped basil

Salt and pepper to taste

**Instructions**:

1. Heat the oil in a Dutch oven over medium-high heat.
2. Stir in the onions and garlic – cook for 6 to 8 minutes until the onions are tender.
3. Add the remaining ingredients and stir well.
4. Bring to a boil then reduce heat and simmer for 20 minutes until the vegetables are tender.
5. Remove from heat and puree the soup using an immersion blender.
6. Season with salt and pepper to taste then serve hot.

## *Chopped Cobb Salad*

**Servings**: 4

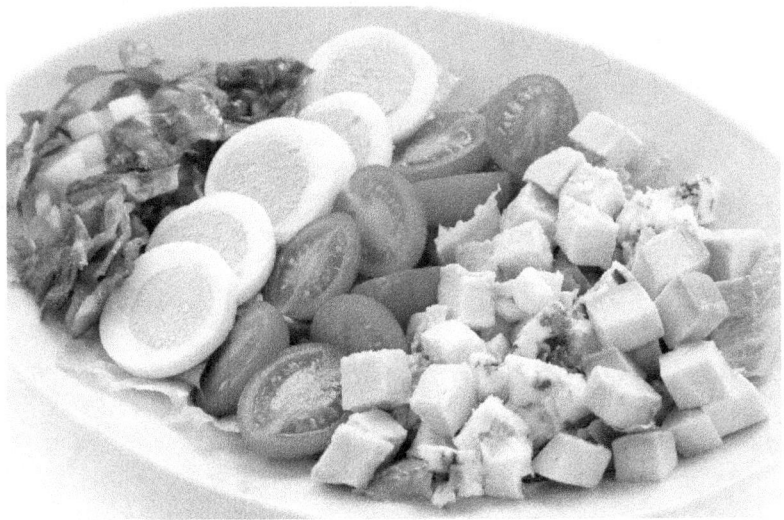

**Ingredients**:

6 cups chopped romaine lettuce

½ small seedless cucumber, diced

4 slices cooked bacon, chopped

2 large hardboiled eggs, peeled and sliced

1 cup cherry tomatoes, halved

1 cup cooked chicken, chopped

½ cup blue cheese crumbles

1 ripe avocado, pitted and diced

**Instructions**:

1. Divide the lettuce among four salad plates.
2. Top the salads with cucumber, bacon, egg, tomatoes, chicken, blue cheese, and avocado, arranging the ingredients in rows.
3. Whisk together the remaining ingredients and serve with the salads.

## *Cream of Mushroom Soup*

**Servings**: 4 to 6

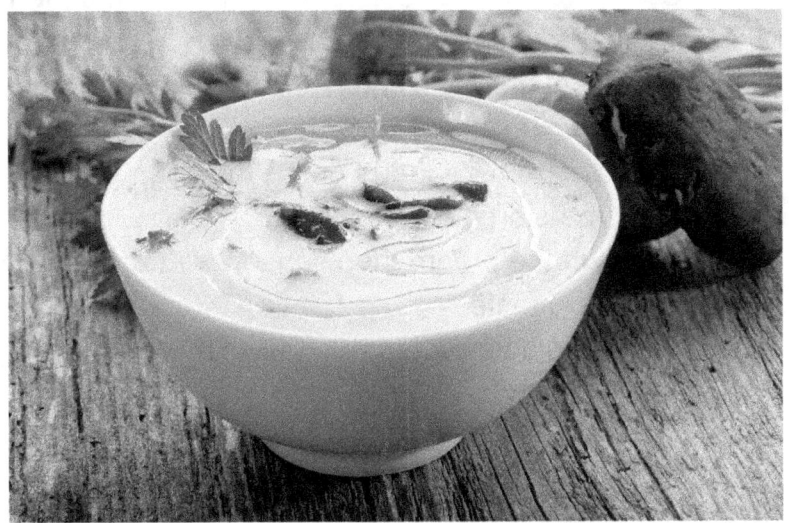

**Ingredients**:

2 tablespoons olive oil

2 lbs. sliced mushrooms

1 cup diced yellow onions

1 tablespoon minced garlic

4 cups vegetable broth

½ cup whipping cream

Salt and pepper to taste

**Instructions**:

1. Heat the oil in a large saucepan over medium heat.

2. Add the mushrooms and cook for 5 to 6 minutes until tender.
3. Set aside 1 cup of the cooked mushrooms then stir in the onions, garlic and broth.
4. Bring to a boil then simmer, uncovered, for 10 minutes.
5. Remove from heat and puree the soup using an immersion blender.
6. Whisk in the cream then season with salt and pepper to taste.
7. Serve the soup hot garnished with the extra mushrooms.

## *Spinach Bacon and Egg Salad*

**Servings**: 4

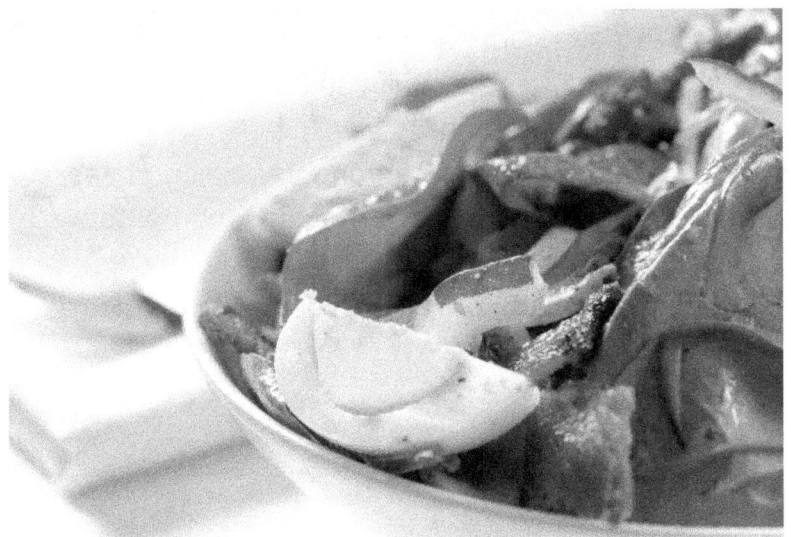

**Ingredients**:

8 slices bacon, chopped

¼ cup red wine vinegar

1 teaspoon white sugar

1 teaspoon Dijon mustard

Salt and pepper to taste

½ lbs. fresh baby spinach

½ medium red onion, sliced thin

4 hardboiled eggs, peeled and quartered

**Instructions**:

1. Heat the bacon in a skillet over medium-high heat until crisp – drain the bacon on paper towels.
2. Whisk the vinegar, sugar, and mustard into the skillet and season with salt and pepper to taste – turn off the heat.
3. Divide the spinach among four salad plates and top with bacon, red onion, and hardboiled egg.
4. Drizzle with the warm dressing to serve.

## *Pumpkin Cinnamon Soup*

**Servings**: 8 to 10

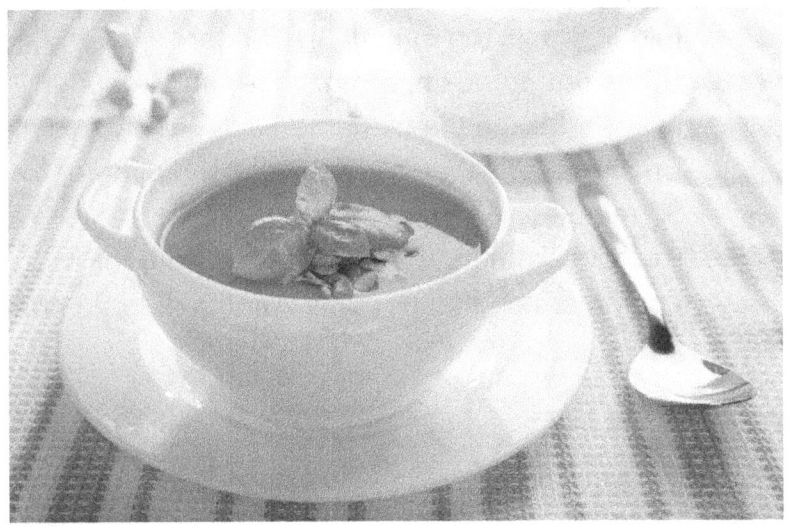

**Ingredients**:

1 tablespoon olive oil

2 cups chopped yellow onion

1 tablespoon minced garlic

2 (15-ounce) cans pumpkin puree

1 (14.5-ounce) can chicken broth

3 ½ cups water

1 (14-ounce) can coconut milk

1 teaspoon ground cinnamon

**Instructions**:

1. Heat the oil in a large saucepan over medium heat.
2. Add the onion and garlic and cook for 5 minutes until the onions are tender.
3. Stir in the pumpkin, broth, water and coconut milk – whisk in the cinnamon.
4. Bring to a boil then reduce heat and simmer for 30 minutes.
5. Remove from heat and puree the soup using an immersion blender until smooth – serve hot.

## *Grilled Salmon with Mango Sauce*

**Servings**: 4

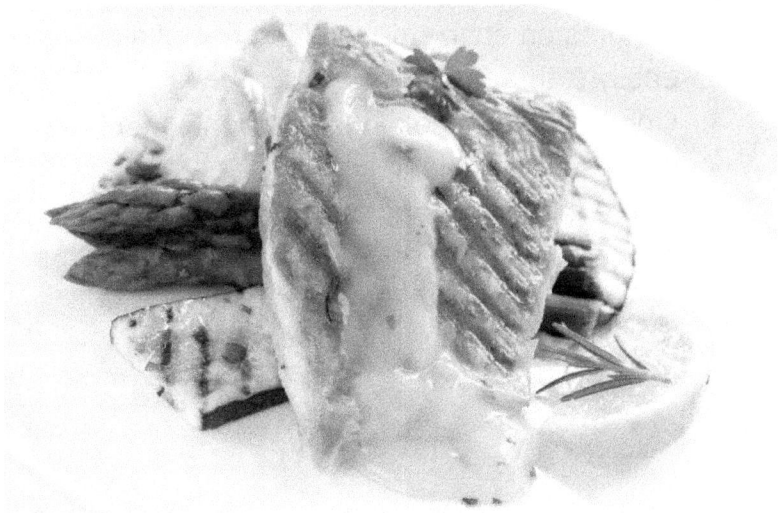

**Ingredients**:

4 (6-ounce) boneless salmon fillets

Olive oil, as needed

Salt and pepper to taste

1 medium ripe mango, pitted and chopped

½ cup canned coconut milk

¼ cup fresh chopped cilantro

**Instructions**:

1. Preheat the grill to medium-high heat and brush the grates with olive oil.

2. Brush the salmon with olive oil and season the fillets with salt and pepper to taste.
3. Place the fillets on the grill and cook for 4 to 5 minutes on each side until the flesh flakes easily with a fork.
4. Combine the remaining ingredients in a food processor and blend smooth.
5. Serve the fillets hot drizzled with the mango sauce.

## *Chicken Cordon-Bleu*

**Servings**: 6

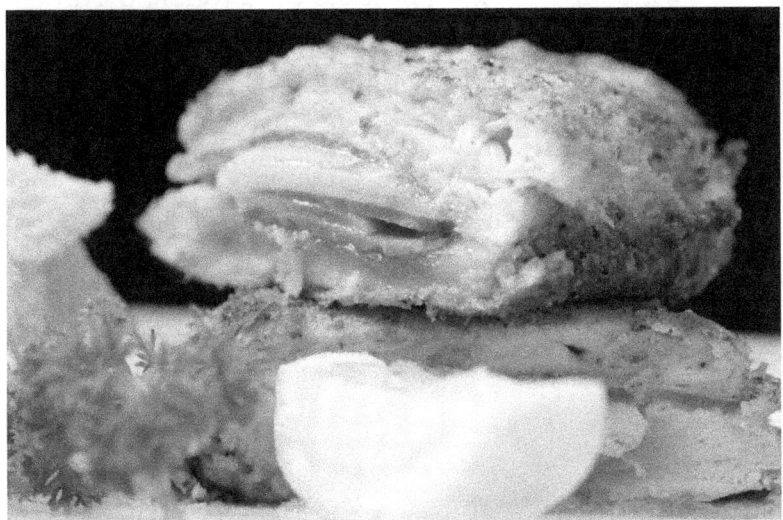

**Ingredients**:

6 boneless, skinless chicken breast halves

6 slices deli ham

6 pieces Swiss cheese

½ cup almond flour

**Instructions**:

1. Preheat the oven to 350°F (180°C).
2. Place the chicken breasts between pieces of parchment paper and pound with a meat mallet until about ½-inch thick.
3. Set the chicken breasts out flat and top each with a slice of ham and a piece of cheese.

4. Roll the chicken breasts up and secure them with toothpicks.
5. Place the chicken breasts on a roasting pan and sprinkle with almond flour.
6. Bake for 35 to 45 minutes until the chicken is cooked through.

## *Grilled Blue Cheese Burgers*

**Servings**: 4

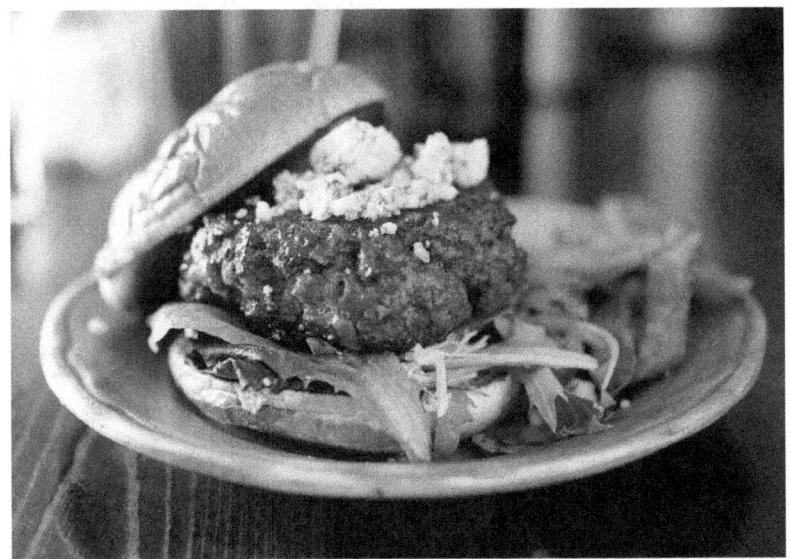

**Ingredients**:

Olive oil, as needed

1 lbs. lean ground beef

¼ cup blanched almond flour

½ cup diced yellow onion

¼ cup crumbled blue cheese

1 tablespoon Dijon mustard

Salt and pepper to taste

**Instructions**:

1. Combine the ingredients in a mixing bowl, stirring well.
2. Divide the mixture into four even-sized patties.
3. Preheat the grill to medium-high heat and brush the grates with olive oil.
4. Season the burgers with salt and pepper to taste.
5. Place the burgers on the grill and cook for 4 to 5 minutes on each side until cooked to the desired level.
6. Serve the burgers on low-carb buns with your favorite burger toppings.

## *Slow-Cooker Beef Bourguignon*

**Servings**: 6

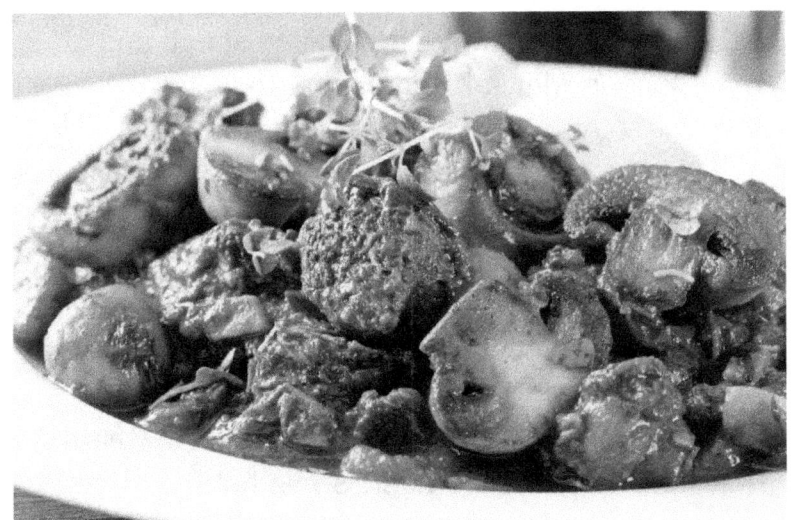

**Ingredients**:

2 ½ lbs. beef stew meat, chopped

1 tablespoon tapioca starch

Salt and pepper to taste

1 lbs. chopped baby carrots

1 large yellow onion, chopped

1 cup sliced mushrooms

1 tablespoon minced garlic

2 cups beef broth

2 cups dry red wine

½ teaspoon dried thyme

**Instructions**:

1. Toss the beef with the tapioca starch and season with salt and pepper to taste.
2. Heat the oil in a large skillet over medium-high heat – add the beef and cook for 2 to 3 minutes until browned.
3. Transfer the beef to the slow cooker and add the carrots, onions, mushrooms, and garlic.
4. Stir in the beef broth, wine, and thyme then season with salt and pepper to taste.
5. Cover and cook for 7 to 8 hours on low heat until the beef is tender. Serve hot.

## *Easy Homemade Meatloaf*

**Servings**: 8 to 10

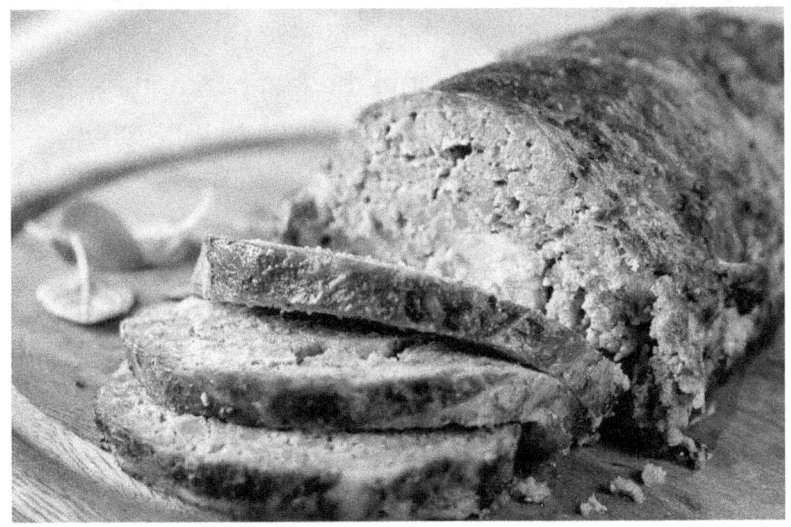

**Ingredients**:

1 ½ lbs. lean ground beef

1 cup plain bread crumbs

1 cup skim milk

1 medium yellow onion, chopped

1 large egg, whisked

¼ cup fresh chopped parsley

1 tablespoon Dijon mustard

Salt and pepper to taste

**Instructions**:

1. Preheat the oven to 350°F (180°C) and grease a loaf pan.
2. Combine the ingredients in a mixing bowl and stir until well combined.
3. Press the mixture into the loaf pan and bake for 50 to 60 minutes until cooked through.
4. Transfer the meatloaf to a cutting board and let rest for 10 minutes before slicing.

## *Chocolate No-Bake Cookies*

**Servings**: about 3 dozen

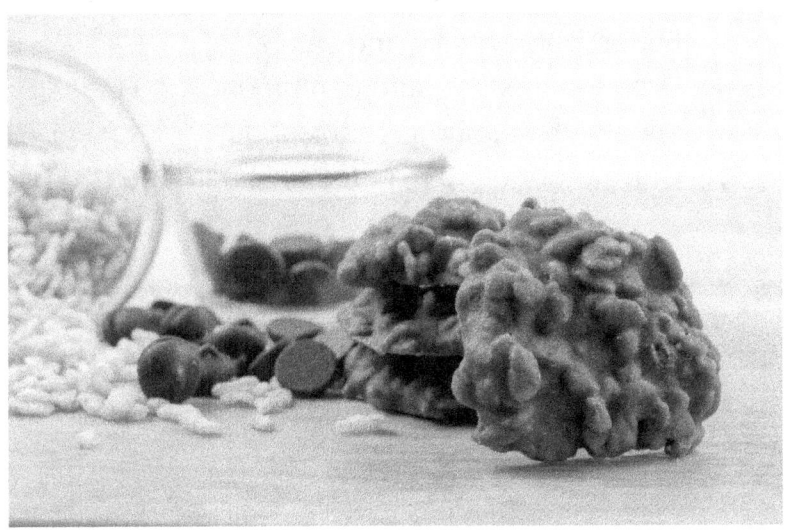

**Ingredients**:

½ cup skim milk

½ cup unsalted butter

¼ cup unsweetened cocoa powder

2 cups white sugar

1 cup peanut butter

2 ½ cups old-fashioned oats

2 teaspoons vanilla extract

**Instructions**:

1. Combine the milk, butter, sugar, and cocoa powder in a saucepan.

2. Bring to a boil and cook for 1 minute until the sugar is dissolved.
3. Remove from heat then whisk in the peanut butter, oats, vanilla and salt
4. Drop the mixture onto parchment-lined baking sheets, using about 1 tablespoon per cookie.
5. Chill for about 30 minutes until hardened.

## *Strawberry Sorbet*

**Servings**: 6

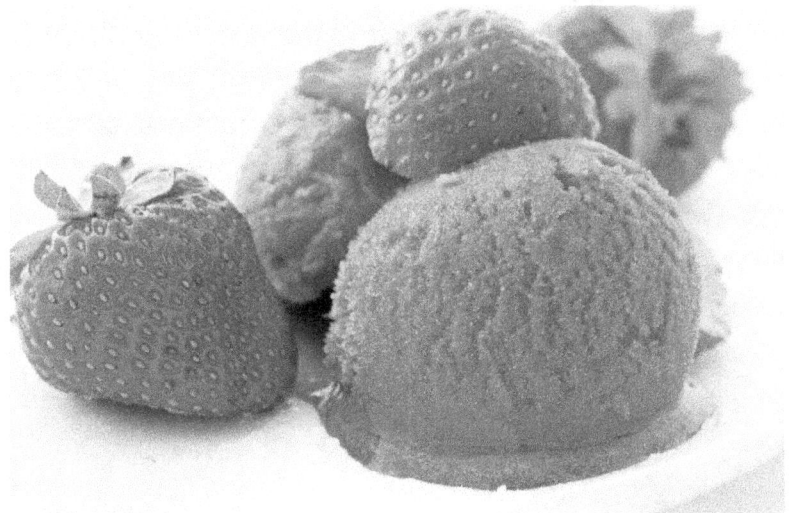

**Ingredients**:

2 ½ cups water

1 ¼ cup white sugar

4 cups sliced strawberries

1/3 cup fresh squeezed orange juice

¼ cup fresh lemon juice

**Instructions**:

1. Whisk together the water and sugar in a saucepan over high heat.
2. Boil for 5 minutes until the sugar is dissolved.

3. Combine the strawberries, orange juice and lemon juice in a food processor – blend until smooth.
4. Whisk in the sugar syrup then cover and chill the mixture for 2 hours.
5. Pour the mixture into an ice cream maker and freeze according to the manufacturer's directions.

## *Avocado Chocolate Pudding*

**Servings**: 6

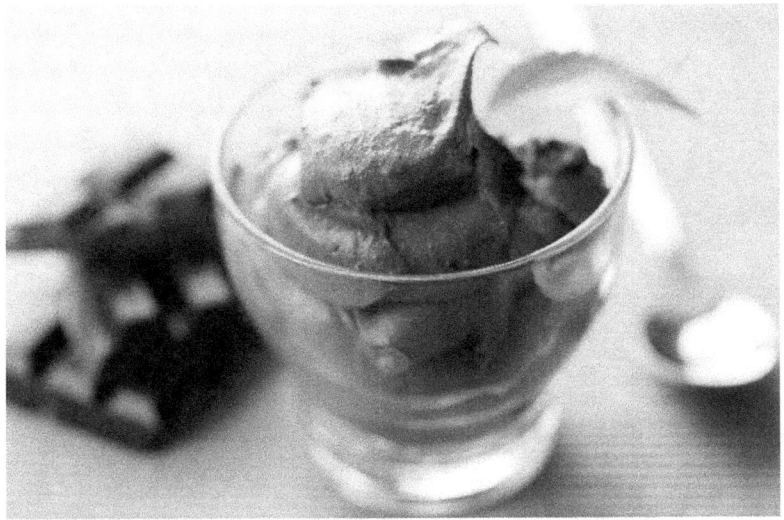

**Ingredients**:

3 medium avocadoes, pitted and chopped

½ cup canned coconut milk

1/3 cup raw honey

1/3 cup unsweetened cocoa powder

1 tablespoon vanilla extract

**Instructions**:

1. Combine all of the ingredients in a food processor.
2. Blend the mixture until thick and well combined.

3.  Spoon the mousse into dessert cups and chill until ready to serve.

## *Meringue Cookies*

**Servings**: about 5 dozen

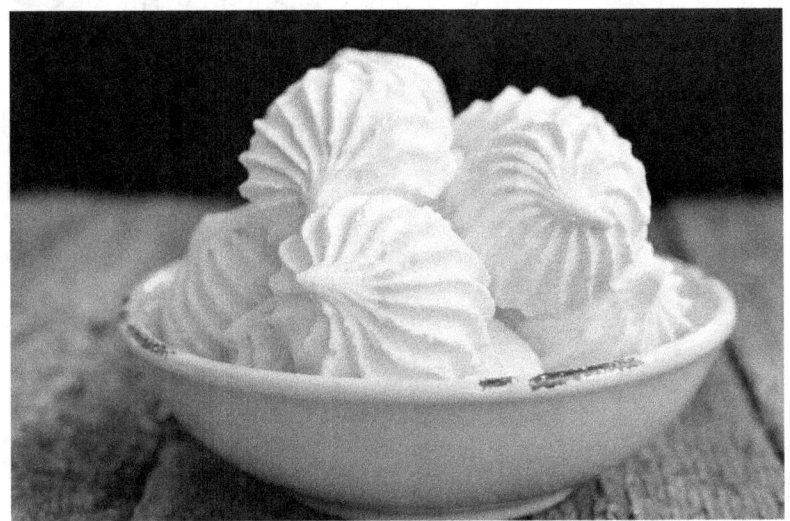

**Ingredients**:

3 large egg whites, room temperature

2 teaspoons vanilla extract

¼ teaspoon cream of tartar

Pinch salt

2/3 cup white sugar

**Instructions**:

1. Preheat the oven to 250°F (125°C).
2. Whisk together the egg whites, vanilla, cream of tartar and salt – beat until foamy.
3. Beat the sugar in, one tablespoon at a time, until it is dissolved.

4. Beat the mixture for 5 to 6 minutes until stiff peaks form.
5. Transfer the mixture to a piping bag and pipe the mixture into 1 ¼ inch cookies on a parchment-lined baking sheet.
6. Bake for 40 to 45 minutes until firm – cool in the oven with the oven off for 1 hour.

## *Cherry Granita*

**Servings**: 8 to 12

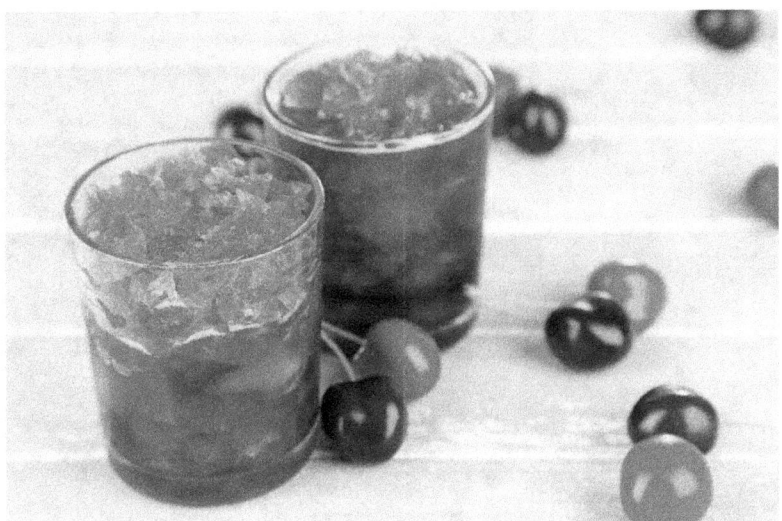

**Ingredients**:

2 lbs. frozen cherries

½ cup white sugar

1 ½ tablespoons fresh lemon juice

**Instructions**:

1. Combine the ingredients in a blender – blend until the sugar is dissolved.
2. Pour the mixture into a square plastic container.
3. Freeze for 6 hours, stirring every hour, until the mixture is the texture of snow.

# Conclusion

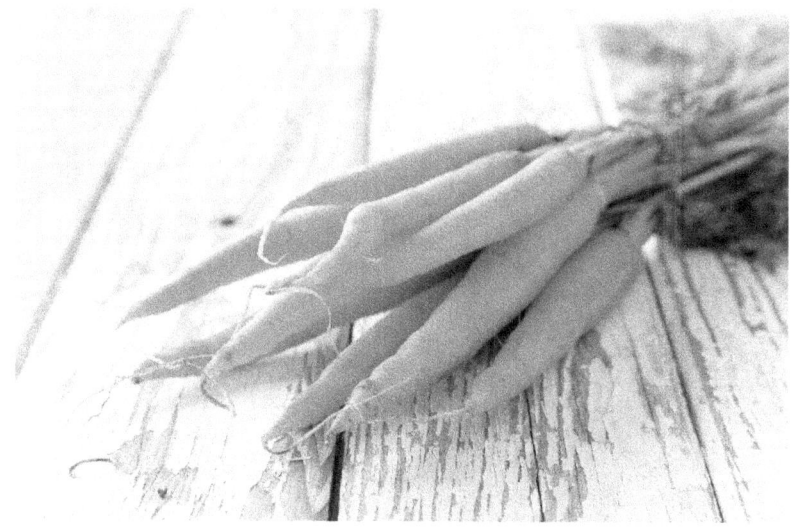

After reading this book, you should have a basic understanding of the Low Carb Diet including a list of foods to eat and avoid. The Low Carb Diet is an excellent tool for weight loss and it is easier to get started with than you might think. If you are ready to give the Low Carb Diet a try this book is the perfect place to start. In addition to receive a quick-start guide to the Low Carb Diet you have also received a collection of delicious Low Carb recipes. To get started with the Low Carb Diet simply pick a recipe from this book and give it a try. You won't be disappointed.